Autism Explained

How an Autistic Child Can Learn to Thrive

In a World That Doesn't Understand

Sara Elliott Price

Published in The USA by:

Success Life Publishing

125 Thomas Burke Dr.

Hillsborough, NC 27278

Copyright © 2015 by Sara Elliott Price

ISBN-10: 1511849800

Disclaimer

Every effort has been made to accurately represent this book and its potential. Results vary with every individual, and your results may or may not be different from those depicted. No promises, guarantees or warranties, whether stated or implied, have been made that you will produce any specific result from this book. Your efforts are individual and unique, and may vary from those shown. Your success depends on your efforts, background and motivation.

The material in this publication is provided for educational and informational purposes only and is not intended as medical advice. The information contained in this book should not be used to diagnose or treat any illness, metabolic disorder, disease or health problem. Always consult your physician or health care provider before beginning any nutrition or exercise program. Use of the programs, advice, and information contained in this book is at the sole choice and risk of the reader.

Table of Contents

Introduction

So your child has autism. For many families this is a devastating diagnosis.

No one wants to be told that their child has autism. However, there is plenty of help out there for families like yours—so don't despair! This book is a great first step, because we'll be taking a look at understanding autism in general and then suggesting practical solutions to meet the everyday challenges of life with an autistic child.

Most likely you've already got a diagnosis for your child. Or maybe you just suspect something's wrong because your child isn't developing in the same way as other children. Maybe you're waiting for an assessment. Either way, as a parent no doubt you have plenty of questions.

Some questions are general: What should I be doing? How can I get help for my child? How will I be able to cope? Others are more specific. How can I get him to talk to me? Why does he scream when he touches certain things? Why does he go into meltdown mode if I have to pick up groceries on the way home from school?

In this book we'll be looking at how to understand the reasons for your child's behavior and practical steps you can take to cope with his disability. We'll help you as you try to help your child understand the strange world he lives in. And we'll offer plenty of suggestions to support you both with the challenges of everyday life.

Chapter 1: Let's Start at the Beginning

Let's start by taking a look at autism. We need to understand what's going on if we're to help our children.

Autism is a developmental disorder – that means it affects the way children relate to the world around them and pick up new skills. It can impact their behavior, social interactions, learning and communication. A child who gets diagnosed at a young age and starts therapy early has the best chance of going on to develop good social skills. However, some slip through the net and don't get diagnosed until they're adults.

There's a wide range of disability within autism, so you could say that no two kids with autism are exactly the same, however they all have symptoms in common. That's why experts call it "the autistic spectrum." Some people have a fairly minor form of the disorder and will be able to lead independent lives. Others are very severely affected and will need lifetime care.

This means that what helps one family may not be so helpful for another – every case is different –but on the other hand there are many other parents going through the same process of learning what works for their child and sharing that information with the rest of us.

Autism facts

According to the website WebMD, about one in every 68 children in the US is on the autistic spectrum – far more boys than girls. Many people with autism have average or higher than average intelligence. Some even have exceptional abilities. However, others have more of a learning impairment, and about 25 percent may never learn to talk in a recognizable way.

Autism affects the way your child sees the world around him. Nothing makes sense to him. Small children with autism can't watch and learn from others, or grasp simple processes and consequences as other little kids learn to do.

People with autism don't like change. What they do like is an ordered world of set patterns, where everything is what it seems and happens the way they have come to expect. They make sense of the world in their own way through rigid routines, all-absorbing interests, and repetitive patterns of behavior.

Autism affects communication, so no matter how much you love your child and sympathize with his isolation it can be very difficult to reach out to him. He may not be able to identify his own wants and needs and tell you what they are or how you can help. He may hate being held or touched.

Someone with autism has trouble understanding other people's emotions or points of view. They can't read faces and don't know when you're upset because they can't see the signs. They may not be interested in other people and they have difficulty in making friends.

People with autism take things literally. They don't understand about idioms, sarcasm, joking, and teasing. They don't get politeness, tact, holding back or "white lies". They say what they think without taking into account who they're speaking to.

Some people with autism are super-sensitive and can react badly to certain tastes, textures, sounds and odors, which seem to be very painful in some way we can't fully understand. So how do you know where your child stands on the spectrum? Well, when your child is referred for an evaluation there is a whole range of psychiatric tests, which make up the assessment. Even though your child may still be very young at the time of the tests, the results will give an idea of the areas he or she will struggle in the most.

Diagnosis is just the start

But that's not the end of the story! Far from it; the diagnosis is only the beginning. The therapies and support your child has can make a huge difference to his progress in the long-term.

And we're not just talking about therapists and pediatricians, but all those who are around your child on a daily basis: parents, siblings, teachers, care workers, grandparents, and friends of the family.

The amount of support from this kind of team has been proven to help children with autism make the most of their abilities and even reach their full potential. Even if it's pretty limited, the therapies and the work the parents do in following through with the treatment can make all the difference.

Do vaccines cause autism?

Some years ago in the UK a then unknown doctor "discovered" a link between autism and childhood vaccines, causing widespread panic. Thousands of parents refused to immunize for years, so children grew up without protection against potentially serious illnesses. Eventually his research was proven to be inaccurate. So no, there is no link between the two.

In the last few years scientists have begun to find out more about the real causes of autism. They've discovered some rare changes in the genes of people who have an autistic spectrum disorder. It's thought that, together with certain other factors, these genetic mutations lead to autism.

But research is still ongoing into what these other factors may be. The age of the parents when they conceive is one possibility, along with certain health problems during pregnancy and difficulties in labor. It's possible that *where the change in the genes already exists* one or more of these other factors may combine with it to cause autism in the child.

It's important that you don't waste time and energy blaming yourself (or anyone else) for your child's autism. It's no one's fault: it's just one of those things. Of course, feeling guilt, anger, despair and frustration are perfectly understandable, and no doubt there'll be plenty of each. But giving in to those feelings and indulging in negative emotions while you wallow in self-pity will make everything harder! Just do your best to acknowledge them and move on.

Sounds tough and unfeeling, right? No, just practical. We've got a job to do – but a big part of caring for your child is looking after yourself, so we're going to be looking at how you can do that too.

Chapter 2: Schedules and Structure

What's the number one thing your child craves? What should be your first priority when it comes to working out how to help him?

Okay, so the clue's in the title. Whether or not your child can tell you – and he almost certainly can't put it into words – a child with autism needs a structured routine.

Most of us enjoy a change from time to time. We like to go away for a break or a vacation. We like to see new places or meet up with old friends. Even at home we like to make changes in our familiar routine or our environment to make a day special, or to improve our surroundings in some way. We might celebrate an anniversary with an evening out or a candlelit supper. We might get new furniture or throw a Halloween party for all the neighborhood kids. You get the picture.

Having a change in routine is good for most of us. It renews our energy and makes us feel refreshed. Even small changes can make a big difference to our mood. But for someone with autism it's the opposite. Change is bad news, and that can be hard for us to understand.

Emergency

But just think about change for a moment. All the changes we've mentioned are positive ones. In fact, we only enjoy a change when it's our choice. Changes without choice tend to be called emergencies! Something goes wrong or breaks down. Someone gets sick or hurt. Maybe worse... Far from making us feel good, they're more likely to involve panic and tears and heartbreak.

Now it's not quite so hard to understand how our autistic children feel. Any changes that come along, even very minor changes are not their choice. Unlike us, they have trouble understanding their world so keeping everything the same is vitally important. And, as every parent with an autistic child has discovered, that often includes every single tiny detail within that routine.

Why is all of this so important? Well, it's about feeling safe. Imagine finding yourself on a strange planet where you have no idea what's going on. Everything seems scary and completely random. You spend all your time trying to make sense of it all, organizing what you can and creating patterns and routines within the chaos just to reassure yourself you're in control. Then as soon as you're beginning to breathe again someone comes along and spoils it all because they fancy a change.

So how can we make our kids feel safe? There are several things we can do to help them establish a sense of security, and they're all very important.

Establish a schedule

This is a priority. Your child needs to have a routine. Draw up a schedule and fix times for meals, therapies, school and sleep for each day. Add in other regular events around these fixed points.

A daily chart is a great start, especially while your child is young, whereas a weekly chart can include details of the different therapies and other regular items like grandparents' visits or shopping trips. Put the chart somewhere where the whole family can see it, like on the refrigerator door. This will become a central feature of your family life; think of it as set in stone, because you can't make changes easily.

Depending on your child's age and ability, he may or may not be able to follow the chart but he will feel the benefit of the routine. Using colors or pictures may help him understand.

Introduce changes gradually

Ideally, as far as your child's concerned, there should be no changes. Ever. But as we know, things will change from time to time. It may be something fairly important, like having the decorators in, or it may be something pretty trivial (to us) like making a detour on the way home from school.

Whatever it is, the process should be the same. Don't introduce change with no warning! Prepare your child well in advance. Tell him what's going to happen several days before and make it sound safe and non-threatening. Keep reminding him in ways that he can understand and praise him for being cooperative.

Be consistent

Part of creating a safe, secure environment for your child is being consistent with him. Okay, you won't always feel like it, but try to treat him the same way every day. Find out about the therapies he's having and continue with the same ones at home. Try to have the school, the therapist and yourself all on the same page.

Your child needs to know that things are the same at home as they are at school and anywhere else he goes. Just as he needs the same routine every day, he wants the reassurance of having familiar objects and people around him who behave as he's come to expect them to. If you can be consistent with his treatment and therapies, and your attitude and behavior, you can create the kind of structured world that makes for emotional security.

Make a safe haven

Your child goes through life being lost and frightened, even though it may come over as being angry and frustrated. He may be happy to accept cuddles and reassurance from you, but he'll probably need a safety zone where he can feel secure when things get too much for him.

Create a safe haven in one room, or even a corner of a room, which your child can escape to. If possible screen it away behind a curtain, or arrange furniture to make it private.

You may not be able to redecorate your whole home, but if possible use the furnishings and décor in this area to make it calm and peaceful. Avoid patterned walls and flooring, and fluorescent lights which some people can hear humming all the time. Use plain, painted walls in neutral colors like cream. A thick rug or carpet makes it quieter as well as cozier, and sensory equipment like fiber optics or soft music can make a soothing environment.

You may need to go through your home to make sure that your child can't reach anything that could do him harm. Safety locks on kitchen cupboards, boxed-in radiators, and childproof containers for medication are all important things to consider. Watch out too for electrical leads and sockets, glass and ornaments.

Your child may not be able to demonstrate affection for you, but never forget you are a very important part of his world. In the next chapter we're going to look at effective ways you can learn to communicate with your child.

Chapter 3: Communication Through Connection

We all know about communication in this modern world of ours. Maybe you've attended seminars on the subject. Maybe you've even given those seminars. And quite possibly you've got all the gadgets and share everything with friends via social media. We certainly know how to communicate in the 21st century.

So now you've got a child with autism and you're struggling with communication. Kids with autism aren't usually able to be sociable and start a conversation or ask questions endlessly like other children, so even if he responds to you it may feel like you're the one doing all the work. It could be that your child can speak quite well, but it's pretty common to have a non-verbal child who doesn't communicate.

Or does he?

A big part of learning about your child is realizing that he is communicating, but most likely in a non-verbal way. When no one understands or people seem to take no notice it's very frustrating for him, and this can lead to tantrums and meltdowns.

In this chapter we're going to be looking at how you can learn to communicate with your child in a non-verbal way, and even encourage him to speak.

Watching for clues

If you ever did that seminar on communication, you'll have heard of the importance of body language when we interact with someone. Being able to read someone's body language is a useful skill to have in business, for example, to make sure you really know what someone's thinking. Of course the reverse is true and you need to make sure your body language is saying the right thing when it comes to winning a contract or getting a job.

The kinds of clues we might look out for in those situations include showing interest by leaning forward and making eye contact, and showing a defensive or negative attitude by crossing the legs or arms. These are all ways of communicating in a non-verbal (and usually unintentional) way.

So what are the clues you should look for in your child? Well, it varies from one to another, so it's a question of learning what happens as he tries to communicate. Watch out for expressions on his face and listen to the sounds he makes as he tries to tell you what he needs. Given time you can learn to "read" him even if there's a language problem, and this will help avoid tantrums of anger and frustration.

But communication needs to go further than just being aware that a meltdown is fast approaching! We're talking about developing a proper relationship.

The four stages of communication

How can we build this relationship? How can we teach our kids to communicate? According to the Hanen Program, a language-development program for children who are slow to learn to talk, they pass through four different stages as they learn to communicate and interact with us. Of course this is generalized and not specially aimed at those with autism, but it's still useful to see the progression.

Stage 1: The "own agenda" stage. The child isn't interested in others but plays on his own. He may use sounds or proper words but they are for his own benefit (because they help him feel calm, for example), not to communicate with others. Most children who have just been diagnosed as having an autistic spectrum disorder are at this early stage of talking.

Stage 2: The "requester" stage. The child has learned that what he says or does has an effect on someone and produces a response. He starts to interact a little and can now communicate by pulling you towards something he wants.

Stage 3: The "early communicator" stage. By this stage the child is using slightly longer interactions with other people. His speech begins to be directed towards others instead of himself, and he may start to echo, or repeat, words and phrases that he hears. Now he will begin to point at what he wants and glance round at you to check your response.

Stage 4: The "partner" stage. The child can communicate at home using proper words and phrases, and can hold a simple conversation. However, in a new environment he is likely to forget his new skills. He may just repeat phrases he's learned by heart instead of really interacting with others. He's likely to forget to take turns to speak, or may seem to ignore the other person altogether. So he'll probably need a little more encouragement until he feels comfortable in the new setting.

Teach your child to communicate

So how can we help our children move along through these stages – especially when they're still at the first one and not interested in communicating or interacting with anyone? It can seem impossible to find a way through the barriers and get close to your child, but it's important to keep trying.

Whatever your child's ability, it's vital to be able to communicate with him. You need to be able to spend time with him, understand what he needs and comfort him when he's distressed. You also need to make yourself understood if you're going to be any help to him as he grows older.

Don't let him just spend hours absorbed in his own world. Remember, you're trying to build a connection between you – an action and response. The aim is for him to learn that it can be fun to do things with other people, and then to learn to communicate and interact with them.

Join in with his activities. Don't wait for your child to invite you, or expect him to come to you for a game. Start from where he is and find ways to join in. If he wants to throw toys on the floor, you could create a connection by picking them up and handing them back one at a time. If he wants to line them all up, you could pass them to him. He then has to interact in turn by accepting your part in the game if he wants to go on playing. Get down on his level so it's easier to make eye contact.

Let him lead. Adults often feel they have to prompt a child to play or suggest a game. In this case you need to follow your child's lead. For example, you could try imitating his noises or gestures and wait for him to notice. Once he does, you have an interaction. The second time it starts to become a pattern, and he may even imitate you in turn. But watch out for signs that he's becoming bored; let him decide when it's time to do something else.

Give things bit by bit. When you give your child a treat or snack, encourage him to ask for more by handing him just a little at a time. Use simple language like asking "More?" so he can pick it up easily.

Make things fun. Playing with your child is more important than teaching, but there's no reason why you can't find ways to make learning fun. Find out what kind of things he likes doing. What makes him smile? What makes him laugh? Let's say it's blowing bubbles. Just blow a few at a time and wait for his reaction. Then blow a few more and ask "More?" After a while you can wait for him to speak or gesture to show he wants you to do it again.

Don't do everything for him. It can be hard to know how much to do for your child as he develops. Try not to do everything automatically; you want him to learn new skills and especially you want him to interact with you by asking for help. However, there's no point in making him frustrated for no reason, so before it gets to that stage show him what to do by breaking things down into very small steps. Don't take it further until he's comfortable doing that step alone.

Give praise and encouragement. Every time you get a positive response or a successful interaction, remember to praise your child. If he imitates you or tries to say something new or learns a new skill, tell him how clever he is. Reinforce good behavior, not bad.

As your child starts to learn a few words, remember to keep things very simple. For example, you could tell him the name of his favorite toys or foods as you hand them to him.

Pictures and photos can be a great help in communicating, because people with autism are very visually oriented. Use them to help your child distinguish between rooms, kinds of foods, contents of cupboards and even to remind him about various people – grandparents, teachers and therapists, for example.

Another way of communicating that some experts recommend is teaching your non-verbal child to sign. While not suitable in all cases, it can be very helpful in the long term. This is something you could discuss with your therapy team to see if it's appropriate in his case.

Chapter 4: A Personalized Plan

In this chapter we're going to look at how you can be proactive and work with professionals to create a personalized treatment plan, based on what you know and discover about your child's strengths and weaknesses.

The way to do this is to become an expert on autism and how it affects your child. Find out all you can about the subject in general (the internet is great for that!). Think about what you notice in your child. What are his interests? What does he do best? What are his weaknesses? Have you noticed any triggers that upset him, or therapies that seem to work and that he enjoys?

IEP or IFSP – what do they mean?

Once your child has been evaluated and tests confirm he has some kind of developmental disorder like autism, a team of professionals meet with you to create an Individualized Education Program (IEP). This program is specially tailored to your child and focuses on getting him the help he will need in school.

In the same way, if your child is under two he will have an IFSP (Individualized Family Service Plan). This aims to work with you and your family to give your toddler the early intervention he needs to help him achieve the best outcome possible.

Your insight will help fill out the therapy outlines put forward by the experts; it will help you contribute to the treatment program and identify areas where he may need extra help. Working with the team in this way will also give you the confidence to continue the therapies at home.

Remember to keep copies of letters and emails from the team treating him. Take notes of details discussed at meetings or over the phone, and write down what you see regarding any changes in his behavior. The idea is that you can build up a file of his ongoing treatment, when it was started and what effect it has on your child. Remember to take the file with you to the doctor or to meetings with the team so you have it to refer to.

Does my child need treatment right now?
Studies have shown that starting therapy early can be very effective in young children. In fact, the earlier you start the better! But even if for some reason you're starting later it can still have a big impact on his future.

What if you're not sure if he has a developmental problem? Doctors would be concerned about a child who doesn't make eye contact, doesn't respond or interact with you, doesn't reach out to be picked up, and doesn't smile, chatter or pay attention to the world around him. Most of these symptoms are noticeable even in babies under a year old, and if you spot any it's wise to get your little one checked out. It's even more important if you notice your toddler is regressing and seems to be forgetting the little skills and interactions he used to have.

Of course, some kids develop and reach certain milestones quicker than others. There may also be times when your little one isn't feeling too good and doesn't want to smile or play. This doesn't mean he has autism, so don't panic. We're not talking about a minute by minute checklist, but a broader view of his development.

You may have to wait to get an evaluation for your child. Because of this delay it's best to get the doctor involved as soon as you're aware there may be a problem. But even if there's a wait to get the professionals' input, you can still begin to help your child.

Working with the professional team
There are a wide variety of autism therapies which aim to correct different problem areas. Some concentrate on treating behavioral and communication issues and improving social skills. Others focus on sensory and movement problems, emotional issues, or food sensitivities.

It's common to have a mix of several treatments to meet the child's needs. For example, your child may have speech-language therapy, behavior therapy or physical therapy. He may need nutritional therapy. He may learn through play-based therapy and occupational therapy. These are all popular treatments.

It's important that you work together with doctors, social workers and therapists to decide on the kind of plan that will help your child the most. It's not a case of either your view or the experts'; it's about combining ideas to make a treatment plan that's just right, and this means you need to be involved from the start.

What can I do?

Think about your child. Before you attend the first IEP meeting, for example, you should prepare in advance by analyzing your child's abilities. If he's able to discuss this, you could ask him what he finds the easiest and most difficult about school.

Do your research and learn what's available and what would be most suitable. Explore the various therapies available, what kind of results they get and whether they might work for you.

Talk to the experts and ask about the therapies they suggest.

They have the experience to be able to advise you. However, you may hear recommendations and suggestions from various people, other parents as well as therapists, who may all contradict each other!

Invite others to join the team. Think about inviting other relatives, supportive friends or helpful professionals to join the team and attend regular meetings. Your child can also be present if this is appropriate for his age and ability.

The website www.helpguide.org suggests you ask yourself these questions when you begin to create a treatment plan:

What are my child's strengths?
What are my child's weaknesses?
What behaviors are causing the most problems?
What important skills is my child lacking?
How does my child learn best (through seeing, listening, or doing)?
What does my child enjoy and how can those activities be used in treatment?

So listen to what the professionals have to say, ask questions and find out as much as you can for yourself. Your child's doctor or pediatrician will be able to help you find out what you need to know about services in your area and how to access them. There is also plenty of information online, including some great sites like autismspeaks.org and autism-society.org.

A good plan

So what does a good treatment plan do? How can you tell if what the experts suggest is likely to work? How can you improve on their recommendations? The website www.helpguide.org sums up the advice from the National Institute of Mental Health. A good plan should:

Build on your child's interests. A great start is to work with your child in the areas he finds most absorbing instead of trying to distract him with more "normal" interests.

Offer a predictable schedule. This gives your child the security of a routine as well as making life easier for you, so aim to have regular hours for therapy.

Teach tasks as a series of simple steps. Learning new skills can be very difficult for children with autism, but breaking the task down into easy steps and mastering each one before moving on makes it much easier to learn.

Actively engage your child's attention in highly structured activities. Your child needs structure in all things, so this is an excellent way to teach him and keep him interested.

Provide regular reinforcement of behavior. A child with autism needs stability and consistency from those around him, so it's important that behavioral therapy is continued at home and school, not just at the therapist's office.

Involve the parents. Parents should be involved in creating the plan for their child, and should also be able to continue with some of the therapies at home. This will reinforce what he learns and greatly increase the hours of treatment he receives.

Remember, there are a lot of therapies and plenty of experts who claim to have your child's interests at heart, but you know your child better than anyone. Your input really does count, so be proactive about getting the help he needs.

Chapter 5: Outbursts, Meltdowns and Repetitive Behavior

As you've no doubt realized, a big part of caring for a child with an autistic spectrum disorder is coping with behavioral problems. Like everything else about autism, these vary from child to child.

Some children are able to understand and accept what's going on, like small changes such as stopping by the store to pick up groceries, and they can express themselves without going into meltdown. Other parents experience a great many problems with their child's behaviors and can be at the end of their rope.

If your child is receiving behavioral therapy, he or she should begin to make progress in this area. But what about in the short term, or if there's a delay before getting therapy – is there anything you can be doing?

In the last chapter we talked about becoming an expert on autism. In this one we're going to look at being a detective. You're going to detect patterns in your child's behavior and try to find the real perpetrator.

Let's take a look at what we can learn about these behaviors.

The website www.helpguide.org/harvard/autism_revolution gives some helpful suggestions based on the book *The Autism Revolution* by Martha Herbert, M.D., Ph.D.

Why does my child act up?

Your child's behavior may make no sense to you, but that doesn't mean it makes no sense at all. There's usually a reason behind everything. Even where there's no logical reason as far as you can see, there's almost certainly either a cause or a trigger. Finding out what they are is a great step forward because you can then work on a way to help your child. Maybe you'll be able to eliminate some of the behaviors altogether.

Obviously some issues are due to things like changes in routine – we already talked about avoiding those wherever possible. Assuming you've already put in place the security of a structured schedule, what more can you do to find out what's going on?

Think again. Instead of looking at your child's behavior as being bad or naughty, change your attitude: something in his environment is upsetting him. The problem doesn't lie with your child but with something else.

We know that people with autism are often hyper-sensitive to all kinds of things – sounds, smells, tastes, textures and visual disturbances. We don't notice these ourselves, but to our children they are very real and seem to cause them intense pain in some way. So some of his behavioral problems may be due to the kind of thing we can't even see. How can we work out what it is?

Keep a log. Start to make a note of what triggers the kind of behavior that seems so inexplicable to you. Write down all the details you can, not just "James did that weird thing again" or "Susie had a meltdown."

What happened just before? What day of the week was it? Try to build up a picture of these behaviors and see if there's a pattern. If so, what's different about that day? There may be a different teacher or a different menu. Try to work out whether the outbursts have something in common – the time of day, the place, and the surroundings. There's almost certainly a trigger.

Look at the environment. Does something or someone near your child set off these outbursts? As well as the kind of stimulus that could lead to over-excitement, or painful sensations affecting his senses, there could be some more obvious reasons for his behavior. Does it happen when an electrical gadget is turned on, for example? Is he reacting to another child's actions or emotions? Is someone rewarding bad behavior by giving him something like a treat – a toy or candy – to keep him quiet?

If the outbursts happen a lot at school, the problem may be social (maybe he fears break times because he has no friends or may even be being bullied), sensory (too much noise, for example) or they could be due to boredom. Talk to his teachers about what's going on at school and what they can do to help. If they seem puzzled, maybe they could also keep a log to monitor these outbursts.

Consider medical causes. Your child's difficult behavior may be due to a physical problem. Watch his body language to see if he could be in pain, and check him over for anything from splinters and stomach cramps to broken bones.

Some behavioral episodes can actually be due to seizures in certain cases. These episodes are usually short, sudden and seem to be unconnected with anything that's happening around him. Watch carefully and note down anything that worries you. Have his teachers noticed anything? Talk to your doctor about what you suspect.

What about a food allergy? Some of the signs are diarrhea within a few hours of eating, and flushed skin on the cheeks and ears. It may be worth cutting out certain foods if you suspect that they trigger an outburst – talk to your doctor about food sensitivities and an elimination diet. Some parents suggest cutting out additives and choosing only natural colors and flavors.

Could it be stress? Your child will be able to pick up on what's going on at home. He may not be able to understand, but he can get stressed out by tension (even though he may be the root cause of most of it!). Exhausted parents, financial worries, siblings acting up... someone with autism can find it very difficult to cope with the normal tensions of family life.

He may also be suffering from anxiety and experiencing a lack of confidence in himself. Again, this is likely to be due to activities outside the home. Some children realize that they can't do the same things as other kids. Some understand that they're different, and this can be devastating. Others may just be struggling with school activities, especially if they're in a mainstream school.

Your child may simply be expressing frustration at his lack of skills or at not being able to make himself understood. Maybe he gets tired, or hungry, or thirsty. Maybe he's scared. Maybe there's just too much information coming at him and he's gone into sensory overload.

What happens next?

So now you've analyzed your child's behavior it's time to see how you can help. You may want to talk to the teacher or the doctor – in fact, this is a good idea if you're worried about his behavior.

You may also have spotted that something in the environment or the daily routine is responsible for upsetting him. Maybe it's just the noise of the refrigerator or the ceiling fan or the fluorescent light, which we barely notice. Maybe there's a physical reason for his outbursts.

Some things are easier to fix than others. No doubt you'll experiment and work out what you can do to improve things for him, but you'll still have a child who's overwhelmed at times and needs to defuse those feelings somehow.

Is there anything we can do to help our kids in this kind of situation? Maybe even avoid them getting overwhelmed? Yes, there is.

Helping your child through sensory breaks

People with autism may experience things differently to the rest of us. Many are over-sensitive to sounds, tastes, odors, textures and visual stimulation. They receive an information overload. Others are under-sensitized to these things, so they don't receive enough information.

Someone with an autistic spectrum disorder may also have trouble with balance and with being aware of their own bodies within their environment. Both of these can make them unsteady and disorientated.

Judy Endow is an adult with autism who has published several books aimed at helping parents and others understand and manage autistic behavioral problems. She suggests creating sensory breaks for your child throughout the day to allow him to release tension and take in the kind of sensory information he needs to relax.

How do we do that? Watch your child and work out (if you don't already know) what repetitive behaviors he likes to do the most. What kind of activity does he choose? Maybe it's something active, like running or spinning. Maybe it's something tactile, like stroking a favorite toy or fabric. Or maybe he prefers a quiet space watching fiber optics or listening to music.

Use his natural choice to create sensory breaks every couple of hours or so (some children may need them more often). Let him have a few minutes of downtime, giving him the chance to regroup and refocus. He can use this time to take in the sensory information he needs which his senses don't supply in the usual way. This information is to reorient himself with his surroundings and may involve physical movement like spinning. It's very helpful in avoiding the kind of situation where he can no longer cope.

These breaks can be used to avoid a build-up of stress and emotion. They can also be used to relieve that stress and emotion once it's already built up. Some people find it's more preventive, others that it's more reactive and they use the time to release some tension. Again, exercise is very useful here. Play a game, take your child for a walk, or if possible let an older one burn up some energy in the gym.

The reason for these sensory breaks is not just to avoid a meltdown, although they should certainly make a difference. Your child needs them to get through the day, much like we might grab a coffee (or even a cigarette) with a sense of relief. It's not the refreshment; it's the few minutes' pause in the midst of our activities. Now imagine those activities involved a load of information coming in from all sides that needed processing non-stop. You surely would look forward to your timeout.

The long-term benefit of creating these sensory breaks is that they teach your child to know when and how to stabilize his emotions and take some time out. They help to teach him self-awareness and self-control.

Next time you see your child doing a repetitive behavior, think for a moment about what he's doing. He's reorienting himself by taking in information about his environment, and releasing tension that he can't express. Is that such a bad thing?

Chapter 6: Creating a Coping Strategy

Being a parent is never easy. Bringing up a child with special needs is going to be tough. Outbursts, tantrums and meltdowns – and that's just your partner! What about the rest of the family? Siblings whose toys get broken or whose friends stay away; relatives who don't understand autism; tensions over finances or disagreements about therapies. How can we cope when it's all so difficult?

Well, no one's going to handle it all the time. There will be days when it's all too much. You might as well accept that now, if you haven't already found it out for yourself.

But all is not lost! What you need is a coping strategy. Here are some suggestions.

Accept your child

It's great to put in place some of the things we've been talking about – to improve your child's behavior and communication, for example – but at the heart of it all is a lost child who needs to be accepted despite his disability. It's easy to lose track of that in the midst of the schedules and therapies, the appointments, the food allergies, the outbursts...

Practice acceptance. Learn to accept your child for who he is. He didn't ask to have autism. He would prefer to be "normal" and happy, but he doesn't have the choice. If you can stop fighting the autism – or him – and accept it, you'll have a calmer and more relaxed outlook on the daily struggle.

Of course, that doesn't mean you should stop all the rest, but sometimes you just need to refocus on the little one in the middle.

Accept yourself
A parent with a special needs child discovers all kinds of things about themselves. Some are good; maybe you've developed a skill for organization and forward planning, or got a taste for research and administration. But some are not so good.

Don't worry, we've all lost our temper or collapsed in tears in the supermarket. We've been tempted to walk away, and of course some parents do just that. But if you're reading this it shows you haven't given up.

You're only human, and there's only so much a human can do. Don't expect too much of yourself, because you're not perfect. You need help, and that means putting in place a support network.

Find a support group

Join an online autism support group and read about how other people are struggling. Exchange useful hints and suggestions, and share the good days and bad days with others who know what you're going through.

You may also find a local group where families can meet up, and this has the advantage of ready-made support within a few miles of where you live. But even if the other members aren't so near, you can arrange visits and meetings as well as loads of phone calls. There are groups too that cater for siblings, helping them share their problems and providing activities and fun events.

Build a network of helpers

Okay, so how are you going to manage if you don't struggle on by yourself? You build a support network of people, that's how! Ideally, of course, these people should live fairly close so you can call on them when you really need them. But even if they're a little further away, they can still be a great help.

These people's role is primarily to support you, not your child – but of course the two areas overlap. Think of a few people you can turn to for help when you need it and talk to them about how their support could make all the difference on a bad day. It may be doing the school run or picking up the groceries. It may be babysitting for an hour or two while you take a nap. It may just be a hug and a little encouragement.

Some of these people may be professionals. For example, you may like to consider getting some counseling for yourself, or talk to your doctor or a local church minister. Others may be friends or neighbors. Don't be too proud to ask – they can only say no!

Get friends and relatives on your side

It's true that often well-meaning relations and friends who know nothing about autism can make things worse. They don't understand why your child ignores them or doesn't behave like other kids. Maybe they resent the attention you give him instead of focusing on them during their visit. Maybe they make hurtful comments.

It's up to you to decide if you want to keep in touch. If it's only a casual acquaintance you could just let them walk away; but if it's your child's grandparents it would be sad to lose contact. The only way round this is to explain (patiently) about autism and what your child can or can't do – both in general terms and what this means on a daily basis.

Some people are scared or self-conscious around people they don't really understand, so try to involve them in some way where they don't feel threatened. Maybe you could suggest a practical way they can help you, or even ask for their advice – say, about fiber optics or additive-free foods. Even if they don't feel comfortable around your child, they can be useful in other ways.

Keep them informed of any progress he makes and let them know how much you appreciate their support and backup, because people who feel they've made a difference are more likely to stay around.

Take a break

There will be times when you need some time out, and it may not be all that difficult to arrange. Do your research and find out about the possibility of putting your child in respite care now and again.

As we know, children with autism don't like change. Respite care is a big change, so this is not something to be undertaken lightly. You may feel it's not worth the trouble. However, with careful preparation it's not impossible, and it would bring you and the rest of the family a much-needed break.

You could also try autism-friendly holidays. Some groups cater for the whole family so your other kids can have fun too, while mom and dad get to relax as well as meet other parents in the same situation.

Take care of yourself

Be sensible and look after yourself as much as possible. Try to eat the right foods and get plenty of sleep at night. You also need time to unwind and relax. Look after your physical and mental health, because if you don't you can't look after anyone else. Don't let yourself get run down or depressed. Get some help.

Putting all these strategies in place will mean you don't have to struggle alone. Talk to your support group and be honest about your feelings. Ask someone for help if you need to. Accept your child and yourself with all the limitations on both sides and just take life one day at a time.

Conclusion

Your child lives in a world where nothing makes sense. Adults with autism speak about how it was as a child: feeling lost, trying to make sense of everything, not understanding other people or their own environment.

So if you can help your child by just bringing comfort and order to his confusing world, you've done all that anyone could ask. You should feel proud of yourself for that alone. All the other subjects we've covered in this book are extras in comparison.

But putting in place some of the other points takes him further: getting him the therapy he needs, finding ways to connect, teaching him to communicate, and helping him learn self-awareness. These are all important steps in your child's journey. He is now on the way to developing vital skills to help him fit into society as he matures.

Using the strategies outlined in this book means you are now well placed to see your child make real progress. You also have a better idea of how you can cope, who you can share with, how to create a support network, what you can do to keep grandparents and friends on board and why you need to take time to look after yourself.

Being the parent of a child with autism is never going to be easy. But these strategies and steps can help you help your child to reach his full potential – and who knows just how far he can go?

Printed in Great Britain
by Amazon.co.uk, Ltd.,
Marston Gate.

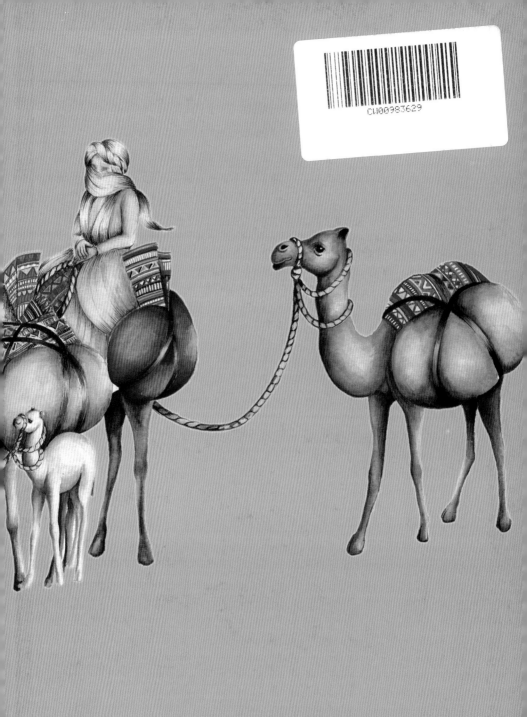

MUSLIM CHILDREN'S LIBRARY

Call to Prayer: The story of Bilal
Author: Edoardo Albert
Illustrator: Angela Desira
Book Design: Stevan Stratford
Coordinator: Anwar Cara
Acknowledgement: Thanks to Assem Kassim for his contribution to image concepts

Published by
The Islamic Foundation
Markfield Conference Centre
Ratby Lane, Markfield
Leicester LE67 9SY
United Kingdom
T (01530) 244 944
F (01530) 244 946
E publications@islamic-foundation.com

Quran House, PO Box 30611, Nairobi, Kenya

PMB 3193, Kano, Nigeria

British Library Cataloguing in Publication Data
        Albert, Edoardo
        Call to prayer : the story of Bilal. - (Muslim children's library)
        1. Bilal ibn Rabah - Juvenile fiction 2. Adhan - Juvenile
        fiction 3. Islamic stories 4. Children's stories
        I. Title II. Desira, Angela III. Islamic Foundation (Great Britain)
        823.9'2[J]
        ISBN-13: 9780860374565

Printed by Proost International Book Production, Belgium

Call to Prayer
The story of Bilal

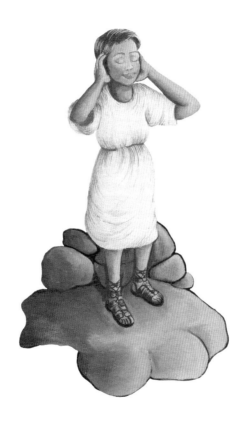

Edoardo Albert

Illustrated by Angela Desira

"No."

The old man's voice was quiet, and yet to the boy's surprise, it filled the glade among the cedar trees.

"That is not correct," he said. "Try again."

The boy took a deep breath, but before he could begin the old man once more said, "No."

"But I didn't say anything," the boy protested.

"Nor could you have," said the old man. He slowly got up from where he was sitting in the shade beneath a cedar tree. They had ridden up into the mountains out of the heat and dust of Damascus in the afternoon, the boy clinging desperately to the old man's waist. He had never ridden a horse before.

Standing beside the boy, the old man said, "Like this," and he began to inhale. The boy watched and it seemed that all the scented air in that little glade among the trees rushed into the lungs of the tall, thin man standing beside him. Then the man exhaled and it seemed as endless as the wind that blew from the sea over the mountains of Lebanon.

"How?... how?" the boy stuttered.

"Not here," said the man pointing to his throat, "nor here," putting his hand on his breast bone, "but here," and he placed both his hands on his abdomen. "This is where the voice comes from." His skin was black against the white of his robe. "But now we will rest for a little while, and you must drink some water, for water is the best medicine for the voice."

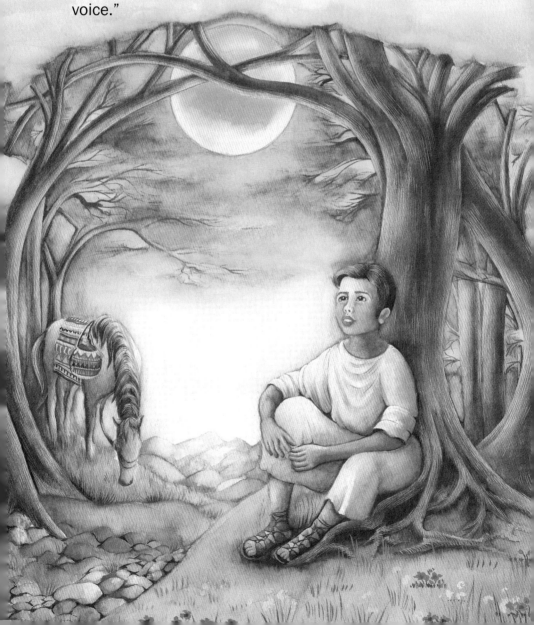

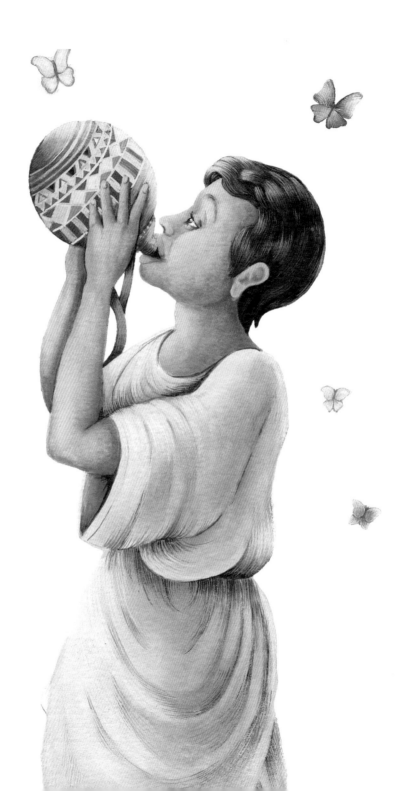

As the old man went to his horse to get the water bottle, the boy decided he would have to ask.

"Master," he said.

The old man stopped and sighed, but he did not turn around. "I am not your master," he said. "You have no master save God," and he took the water bottle from the saddle bag.

"Are you really Bilal, son of Rabah?" said the boy in a rush. Then he stopped, shocked at his own courage. The old man halted. Finally he turned to the boy who stood in the clearing, not quite daring to look at the old man who had bought his freedom just a few weeks ago.

"I am only a black man who until yesterday was a slave," said the old man. "But the answer to your question, Saeed, is yes. I am Bilal, son of Rabah, and like you I was born a slave. But now, drink."

Saeed, who had never in his whole life been given the first drink, barely moistened his lips and would have given the bottle back, but the old man again told him, "Drink."

The bottle was nearly empty before Bilal would accept it. As the old man raised it, Saeed, who grew more courageous by the day, blurted out, "Master, please, will you tell me of your days with the Prophet? You were with him, you knew him, what was he like?"

Bilal looked at the boy. "It is not my wish that people should know of my past, Saeed," he said. "For once they know, they will all come to me and beg me to make the call to prayer again, and that I will not do. So you must promise to keep your peace and not talk of this to the other boys. Do you promise?" Bilal stooped down and gazed into the face of the boy.

Seeing his own reflection in those dark eyes, Saeed thought that once they would have held the reflection of Muhammad, the Messenger of God. He could not speak, but only nod.

"Sit down, then," said Bilal, "and I will speak."

The old man and the boy stretched out in the shade beneath the trees, and Bilal's gaze turned inward, to the book of memory. For a while he was silent, and the only noise came from the cicadas. But then in a quiet voice Bilal began to speak.

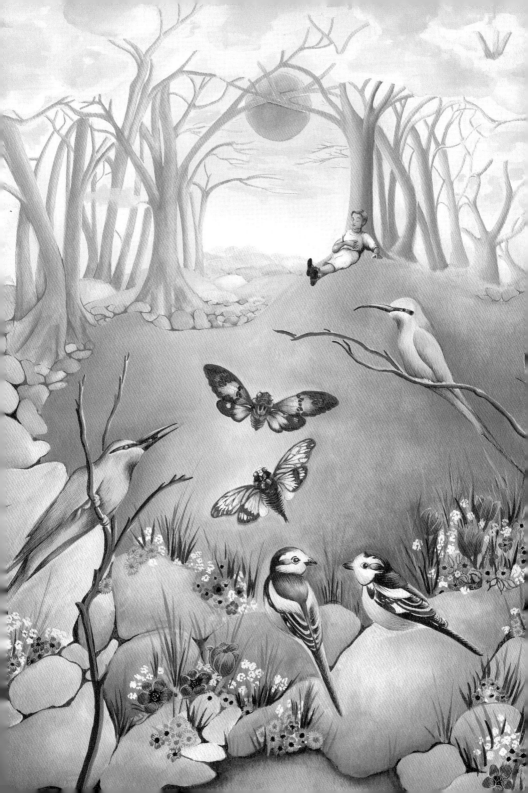

"You ask me what the Prophet was like, and in truth that is not a question I can answer. I do not have the words. But if you read the Book, then you will know what the Prophet was like, for he is there, within its pages."

"Yes," said Saeed, nodding. "Master, is it true that you were a slave and your master crushed you under a rock when you became a Muslim and that you made the first call to prayer and..."

"And enough," said the old man, but he could not help but smile at the boy's eagerness.

"What you say, Saeed, is all true. I, Bilal the Ethiopian, was born a slave, the son of slaves. But it is most strange that when I gave away the one thing that belonged to me, when I gave away my heart, then I became free. For in submitting to God there is freedom from the fear of any man."

"Even your master?" asked Saeed, who until recently had been a slave and was not yet truly free.

Bilal smiled, but it was a smile touched by pain. "Even him," he said. "Even Umayyah bin Khalaf. The slave, Bilal, no longer feared his master. Maybe that was why he so hated me."

"Is it true what they say he did to you?" asked Saeed.

"And what do they say?" asked Bilal.
"They say he staked you out on the ground in the midday sun and put huge rocks on your chest."

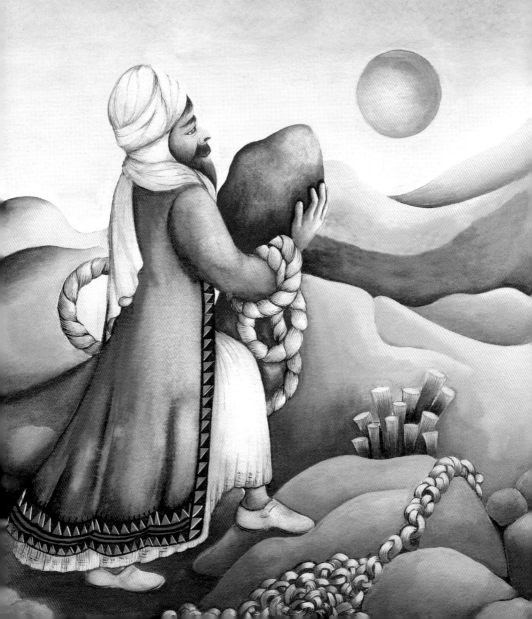

"That is true," said Bilal. "You cannot know what it was like in those days, Saeed. The Ka'ba itself was full of idols. Can you imagine it? But, no, do not even try. When I first heard it whispered that a Prophet had arisen among us, proclaiming there is but One God, oh, it was like sight to my eyes and hearing to my ears. I was a slave, uneducated, thinking the wise worshipped all these gods, so who was I to think it wrong? Then the whisper, like the first wind before dawn, flowing through the streets of Makka. One God. One God. One. And I believed. My bones knew it to be true. I believed, and my master hated me for it. Since I was just a slave and had no one to protect me, Umayyah thought to crush me."

The old man paused and smiled thinly. "But maybe in trying to destroy me beneath those rocks, my master gave me a great gift. For that was when I truly learnt how to breathe."

"But how did you breathe with the rocks crushing you?" asked Saeed.

"Exactly," said Bilal. "Maybe you would like to try and you will see that the only way to breathe when being crushed is from the abdomen, from the true dwelling place of the voice. Umayyah bin Khalaf gave me my voice, and I first used it as he whispered the names of his idols in my ear. I used my voice to call on the One God. I called it out, in the face of my master, in the faces of Quraysh. One God."

Bilal fell silent for a while and the boy was about to speak when again the old man looked at the boy. "So, you see, if you want to make the call, you must do those breathing exercises."

"I will, I promise," said Saeed. "But how did you escape from Umayyah?"

"I did not escape," said Bilal. "I was bought and then freed by such a man that it was an honour to be bought. For it was Abu Bakr, the Companion of the Prophet and the first Caliph who freed me, but I was merely one of his many good deeds. My master was a greedy man, and when Abu Bakr came to him and offered to buy me, his greed overcame his hate and I was sold for the last time."

"Is it really true that you were the second man to enter Islam after Abu Bakr?" asked Saeed, for he had heard so from some people, although others said different.

The old man smiled. "No, that is too great an honour for me, Saeed. But say instead that no one came from lower than I, for I was buried beneath a stone, and I was lifted up."

Bilal bent his head and was silent and the boy did not dare to speak.

"They hated us," Bilal said, looking up at Saeed. "The Makkans hated us, for we were a threat to their gods but more importantly we were a threat to their

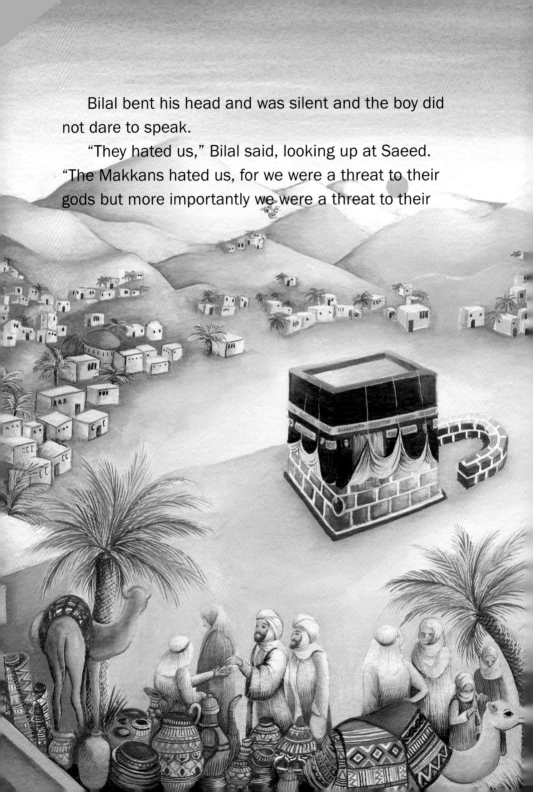

trade, and they were greedy people. Even when I was free, they persecuted me, they persecuted all of us, but most of all they persecuted the Prophet. So we left." The old man smiled. "Our leaving was the

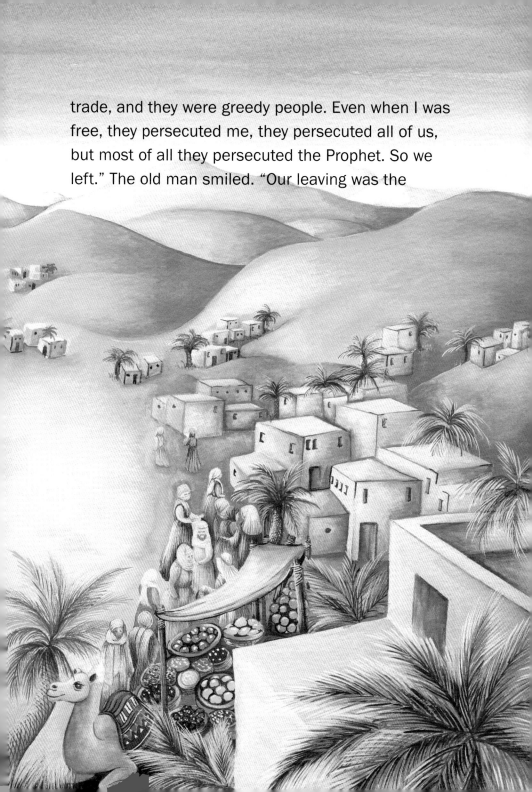

beginning, for that is when history starts. The Hijrah. The first year of a new world. Though I must admit I did not realize it when I was stumbling with the others through the desert on my way to exile in Madina."

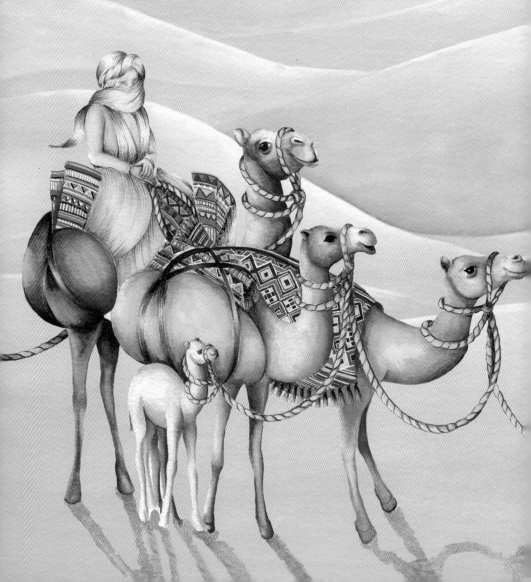

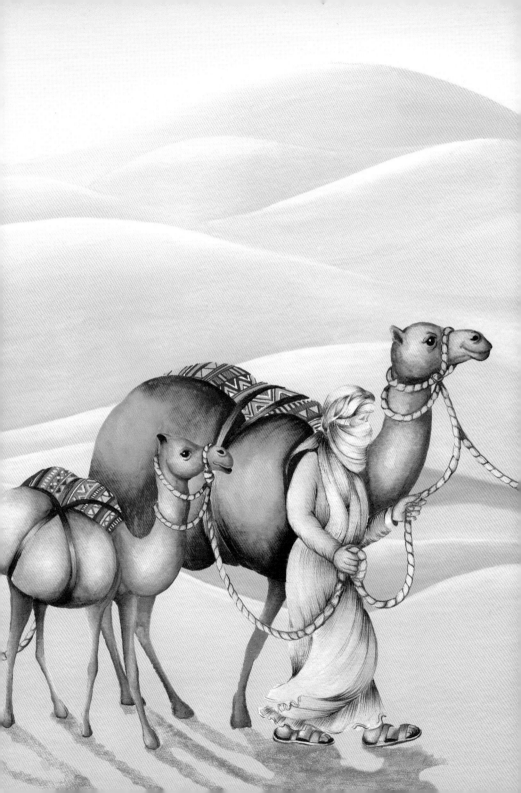

At the mention of Madina, Saeed grew even more excited. He had his arms round his knees as he sat on the ground and he pulled tight on his legs. Bilal's face remained solemn, but there was a smile in his voice when he said, "Soon it will be time for you to start your work again. Ask now, if there are any questions in your heart."

The boy suddenly looked terror-struck. No one had ever put him on the spot and asked him if he had any questions before. Bilal saw the expression on his face. "I am sorry, Saeed," he said. "I should know, a slave does not question, he listens. But you are no longer a slave, and you must speak. What do you wish to ask?"

Saeed swallowed. How could he ever hope to make the call to prayer if he could not even ask a simple question?

"How... how did the Prophet ask you to make the call?" he said finally.

Bilal nodded. "You should know this," he said. "The first time the call was heard was dawn in Madina, when I, Bilal, who only yesterday had been a slave, stood on the highest rooftop near the mosque and called all the faithful to prayer. And they came. They came not to the sound of horns or the wooden

20

clapper – the *naqus* – but to the sound of a voice, calling them. For in the night 'Abd Allah ibn Zayd had come to the Prophet and told him of a dream."

"But what happened in the dream?" asked Saeed.

Bilal's smile grew broader. "See how easy it becomes to ask," he said. "And easy to answer, for in his dream 'Abd Allah ibn Zayd saw a man dressed in green carrying a *naqus* and he asked to buy the *naqus* from him that it might be used to call the faithful to prayer. But the man dressed in green taught him a better way, and it was taught to me, and now I teach you, Saeed."

The boy sat back. For the first time he realized a part of what he was being shown to do.

"Each morning," said Bilal, "I would climb up onto the roof before dawn and wait there for daybreak. It was so quiet. And sometimes," he smiled, "so cold. I would then pray to God, asking His help for the Quraysh that they might accept Islam. Then I would stand and make the call to prayer."

The old man smiled at the memories. He was talking more than he was accustomed to, but the boy's questions had drawn sweetness from the wells of his mind.

"Ah, Madina of blessed memory," he said. "For in Madina the Prophet gave me a wife." The old man paused. "Do you know the story?" he asked.

"No," said Saeed, "no I don't."

"Then I will tell it, for it shows much of the Prophet and, I pray, a little of me. 'Abd ar-Rahman ibn 'Awf went to the Prophet when he was sitting in the mosque and asked him to suggest a suitable husband for his sister. The Prophet said my name. Sometimes I like to imagine the expression on 'Abd ar-Rahman's face when he heard the name Bilal, for his was one of the wealthiest and noblest families of Makka and here was the Prophet suggesting his sister marry a freed black slave. Such things had never happened before. But whatever the expression on 'Abd ar-Rahman's face, he made no reply and left," Bilal explained

"Then, a few days later, 'Abd ar-Rahman again went to the Prophet and asked him the same question. The Prophet said my name again but 'Abd ar-Rahman made no reply and left. It was the third time, a few days later still, when 'Abd ar-Rahman received once more the same answer to his question that he said, 'Messenger of God, my sister will be happy to be the wife of a man you hold in such regard.' But still there were some relatives who were not satisfied with a slave as a member of the family and they went together to the Prophet to ask for his surety on my behalf."

The old man paused. "I have heard this from many people and I pray that it is true, for they tell me that when the Prophet heard them ask for his surety, he grew angry and said, 'Who are you to question Bilal ibn Rabah, who are you to question a man of paradise?' But these old ears did not hear those words spoken and I never dared ask the Prophet if what people said was true. And that is how in Madina I gained a family." The old man smiled at the boy.

"But why did you leave Madina?" asked Saeed.

"I could not stay," said Bilal. "Not after the Prophet died. Each dawn I would be the one to wake him as I went to make the call. I went everywhere with him. I was his steward in battle and I was his servant in peace, Saeed. Some people said it was well that I am black because I was like the Prophet's shadow. And how can a shadow remain after its object has gone? I could not stay in Madina after he died. So I came here to Syria." The old man smiled ruefully. He looked up at the sky. The sun was getting low. It would not be long before it set.

"Have you any more questions, Saeed?" he asked. "It is time you got back to work."

"Did you ever make the call after the Prophet died?" asked Saeed.

The old man looked into his treasury of memory. "I have done so twice," he said. "Once when the Caliph Umar conquered Jerusalem. And the last time, when I went to visit my friends who still remain in Madina. While I was there the two grandsons of the Prophet, Hasan and Husain, asked me to make the call. How could I refuse? So these old legs again walked up the steps they had walked so many times before, and I stood looking over the roofs of Madina.

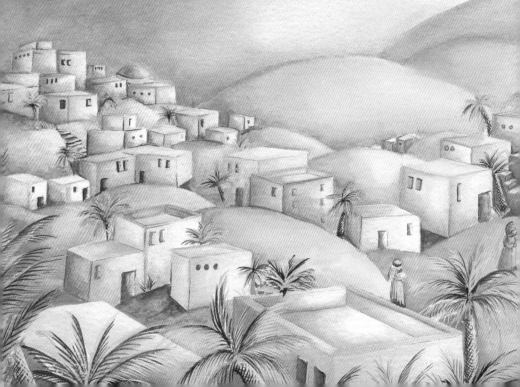

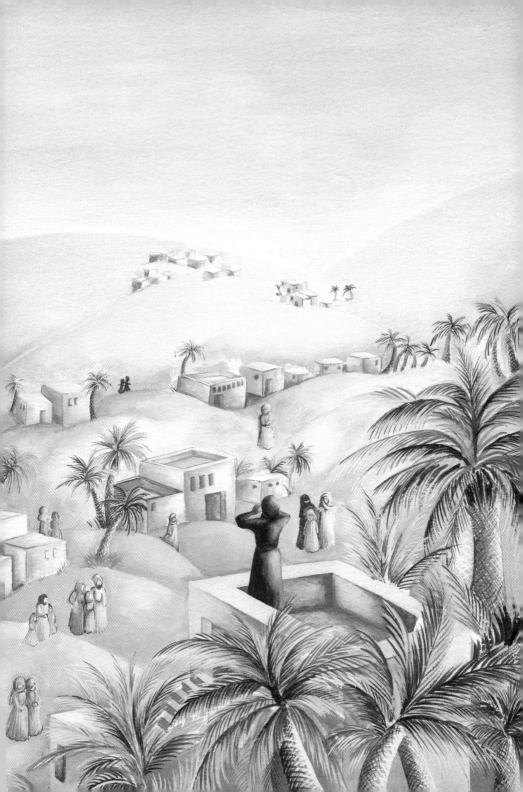

Then my eyes became blind with the tears I began to shed, but my voice was still strong and I called out, 'God is Most Great.' I was told afterwards that the people stood transfixed with the memory of the Prophet when they first heard my voice. When I called out, 'I testify there is no god but God' they tell me that the people began to weep. And when the people heard me call out, 'I testify that Muhammad is the Messenger of God', I was told that they came rushing out into the streets, convinced that the Prophet had returned. But it was only old Bilal, alone and crying the tears of an old man's memory."

Bilal looked at the boy. "I will not make the call again, Saeed."

"Will you teach me?" asked Saeed.

The old man laughed and got to his feet. His knees hurt but he did not let that show. "Of course," he said. "That is why we are here. Now come, stand before me."

Bilal put his hands on the boy's shoulders and bent his face to the boy's.

"When you make the call, remember what you are saying. These are the most important words any man can hear. You are calling him to salvation. Let no man say on the Day of Judgement that he did not come to prayer because he could not hear or understand you."

Saeed nodded, his mouth suddenly dry. He wondered if he would be able to speak at all.

"Remember the mouth and the throat are just the doors to the dwelling place of the voice. Remember the vowels carry the words and the consonants shape them. Remember all these things, but remember what you are saying most of all, Saeed. Now come."

And the old man led the boy to the edge of the clearing. Together they stood looking down the slopes of the hills to the towers and walls of Damascus, stained red by the setting sun. The birds and insects were quiet. The world was waiting.

Bilal turned to the boy at his side.

"Make the call, Saeed," he said.

And in clear high tones that rang from the rocks and reflected off the hills, the boy called:

"God is Most Great. God is Most Great.
God is Most Great. God is Most Great.
I testify that there is no god but God.
I testify that there is no god but God.
I testify that Muhammad is the Messenger of God.
I testify that Muhammad is the Messenger of God.
Come to prayer. Come to prayer.
Come to salvation. Come to salvation.
God is Most Great. God is Most Great.
There is no god but God."

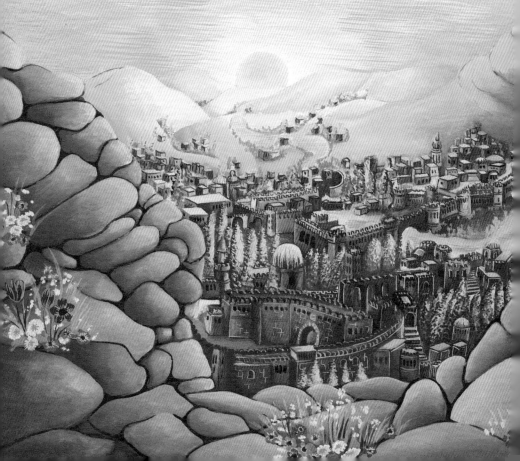

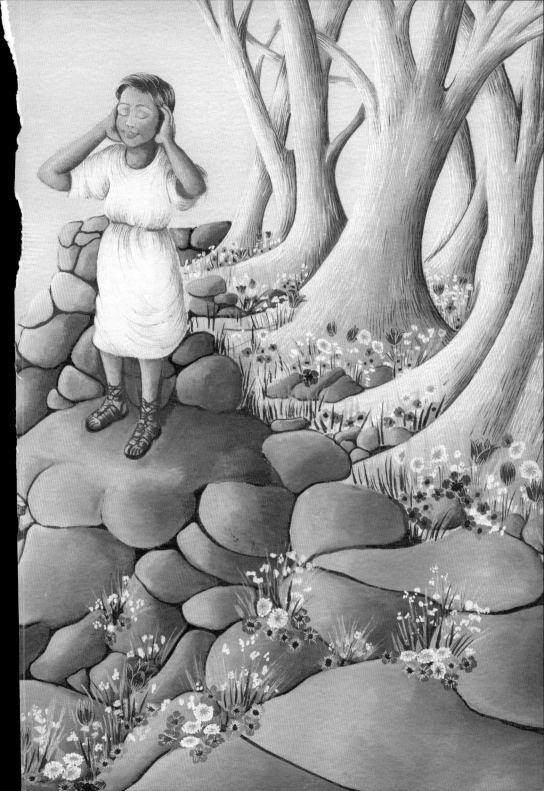

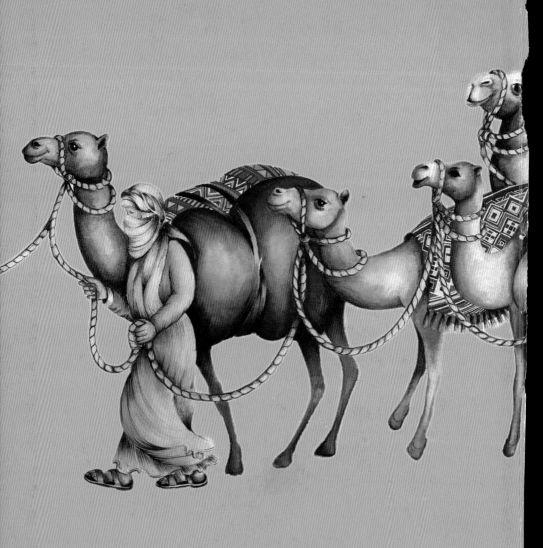